Fad Diets Explained

Everything you need to know about

America's top 15 diet plans

Fad Diets Explained

Everything you need to know about

America's top 15 diet plans

Sam Walker

Fad Diets Explained
Everything you need to know about America's top 15 diet plans

Edited by HITE Publishing Co.
Published by HITE Publishing Co.
United States of America

Electronic Edition: October 2015

Table of Contents

Introduction

Sooner or later, most of us start thinking about a healthy diet. The reasons for it may be different: to lose weight, to improve cholesterol ratio, to decrease heart disease risk, or just to improve mood and higher our energy levels. Healthy nutrition has always been an answer to make key question of a human's well-being.

Whichever reason you have, the difficulties start the same moment when you make a decision to start your diet, because the first question you have to answer is "Which diet should I choose?" If you start searching on the internet, you will find hundreds (if not even thousands) of them, but... how reliable is this information?

You can also talk to your doctor, which is an absolutely good idea (and you do have to do it before starting a diet), but how well does a doctor know your tastes and individual preferences?

To make your choice easier, we have carefully selected the best diets that had been popular during the last years, and which, according to the dieters' feedback, had brought the most effective results and significantly improved their health. Besides that, we have also analyzed the opinions of the specialists and professionals in the field of dieting and nutrition, in order to make sure that achieving your dieting goals will be safe and healthy.

This book includes an overview of 15 diets: The Zone, Atkins, South Beach, Paleo, Mediterranean Diet, Mayo Clinic Diet, DASH Diet, TLC Diet, Weight Watchers, Jenny Craig, Biggest Loser, Slim-Fast, NutriSystem, Vegetarian Diet and Raw Food Diet.

The book gives an objective opinion and facts about the pros and cons of each of them, explains its origin, describes how it works, which results it may bring, what are its potential risks, how easy to follow the diet and what are the approximate costs for each of them.

It is my sincere hope that it will be useful and helpful on your way of dieting and healthy nutrition!

1. The Zone

Ranking: 3.9 out of 5.0

How Long It's Been Around

The Zone diet was developed by Barry Sears. Sears has a Ph. D. in biochemistry, but no special training in nutrition. He began working on this diet in the 1970s. After his father died prematurely of a heart attack at age 53, Sears began studying the role of fats in the development of cardiovascular disease.

In 1995, his book Enter the Zone, became a bestseller. Since then he has written a dozen books and cookbooks about the Zone diet, established a Web site, and developed a program of home-delivered Zone meals, turning the Zone diet concept into a multi-million dollar business.

How It Works

The Zone diet is designed to promote fat loss and weight loss, but its developer also claims that the diet brings about substantial health benefits. This diet is highly structured. Participants in the Zone diet are instructed that every meal and every snack should consist of 40% carbohydrates, 30% protein, and 30% fats.

This produces what Sears considers the ideal ratio of protein to carbohydrate. The protein to carbohydrate ratio of .75, Sears says, allows the body to function at optimal level. He refers to this optimal functioning as being "in the Zone."

Being in the Zone claims TO boosts energy, delays signs of aging, helps prevent certain chronic diseases and allows the body to function at peak physical and mental levels. The Zone diet is less concerned with people reaching a specific weight than with reducing body fat. The goal is for men to have only 15% body fat and women 22% body fat.

The amount of food a Zone dieter consumes is based on that person's protein needs. Protein needs are calculated based on height, weight, hip and waist measurements, and activity level. The amount of carbohydrates and fats allowed on the diet derives from the calculation of protein needs. The result is a daily diet that usually ranges from 1,100–1,700 calories. Dietitians consider this a low calorie diet. To simplify meal planning, portions of proteins, carbohydrates, and fats are divided into Zone Food Blocks. Instead of eating a certain number of calories, the dieter eats a specific number of Zone Blocks in the required proportions.

Expected Results

The developer of the Zone diet Barry Sears says that following the Zone diet it is possible to lose 1-1.5 lb (6-7 kg) per week. It guarantees permanent weight loss, improvement of mental and physical state. It also prevents chronic cardiovascular diseases, improves immune system functioning, decreases signs of aging and increases longevity.

Weight loss is often the goal for people on the Zone diet and, in the short term, weight loss is achievable. Long-term claims that the diet can reduce heart disease and diabetes risks have not yet been supported by research.

In a study that compared the nutritional elements of the Zone diet with 15 other popular weight-loss diets, the Zone ranked as one of the top five, tied with the diet based on the U.S. Department of Agriculture's Food Pyramid. The Zone diet is a popular, high-protein diet that can yield weight-loss results, although you may have to pay attention to overall nutritional requirements while following it.

Health risks/ Dangers

No indications of serious risks or side effects have surfaced. The plan is generally safe for everyone. However, if you have a health condition, check with your doctor to ensure the Zone diet is right for you.

How Easy It Is to Follow

The Zone diet it is relatively easy to follow as soon as you are aware of which foods you have to to limit. If you make sure each meal contains the necessary percentage of carbs, protein, and healthy fat can be tedious. Some people may find Zone's strict eating schedule – breakfast within one hour of waking up, and then snacks and meals every five hours – daunting.

Recipes are available, though ensuring meals conform to the 40:30:30 rule could prove time-consuming. Dining out is doable. The company's online and printed resources may be helpful. Sears' book *A Week in the Zone* offers breakfast, lunch, dinner, and dessert recipes, as well as snack ideas. Choices range from chicken fajitas to seafood salad. Eating out is allowed as long as you ignore the bread basket, choose a low-fat protein entrée, and order vegetables instead of starches and grains. Once your meal arrives, examine the size of your entrée. If it's larger than your palm, plan to take some home.

There are some restrictions regarding alcohol, since beer and wine contain carbs, and all alcoholic drinks add some calories. However, you can still consume alcohol, but in moderate portions. The experts suggest two drinks a day for men and one for women. According to Sears, the best choice would be red wine, since it's packed with polyphenols, antioxidants that purportedly thwart inflammation and other health problems.

In order to save some time, you can purchase online the Zone 1-2-3 foods. These products are not full meals, but rather individual dishes, such as cookie, pasta, pizza, etc. Each item contains 1 gram of fat for every 2 grams of protein and 3 grams of carbohydrates. This ratio will suppresses your appetite for some time, up to six hours.

They are not required, but can make the general flow of your diet much easier. Moreover, if you purchase Zone 1-2-3 foods, you will get connected with a Zone Coach, whom you can contact in order to get some support and motivation that will also lead you to the better results and make your experience much easier. Besides that, the coaches will also give you some practical tips and advices on healthy eating and dieting.

There is also an opportunity to get the online membership at zonediet.com. It is free and gives you an access to a body fat calculator, recipes, monthly newsletters, podcasts and videocasts on the topics of health.

Another good thing about the Zone diet is that you will not feel hungry. On the Zone diet you need to have regular snacks, so in fact, you will not stay more than five hours without food, which will keep your blood sugar from dropping and hunger pangs from striking. And also, which not less important, the Zone diet's recipes are tasty, so you don't have to exclude from the menu your favorite pancakes, meat, cheese or wine. You can even allow yourself some extras, as long as it doesn't happen every day, and you can still come back to the diet after. These are the benefits of the diet that are making it quite easy to follow for everyone.

Price/ Cost

Online membership is free. Supplies of the Zone 1-2-3 foods for a week may cost about $70. A package that consists of 14 shakes will cost about $35. A book "A Week in the Zone," which will guide you through the diet, costs $7.99, and another one, "The Mediterranean Zone," is $20.

2. Atkins

Ranking: 2.3 out of 5.0

How Long It's Been Around

The Atkins diet is named for Robert C. Atkins, M.D., the diet's founder. Dr. Atkins introduced his Diet Revolution in 1972. From the beginning, Dr. Atkins, a cardiologist, said that limiting intake of carbohydrates (sugars and starches) would improve health and aid in weight control. The original premise for developing the diet came about because of Atkins' frustration with the increasing rates of obesity and chronic diseases such as diabetes.

How It Works

You go through four "phases," starting with very few carbs and eating progressively more until you get to your desired weight. Keeping carbs at bay isn't as simple as saying No to sugar and baked potatoes. You'll keep acceptable foods lists handy and polish your arithmetic skills. In phase 1, for example, you're allowed 20 grams a day of "net carbs" (pull out the food list), 12 to 15 of them from "foundation vegetables" (pull out another list) high in fiber. But as for fat, you don't even have to trim it off your steak.

Throughout the diet, Dr. Atkins recommended drinking at least eight 8-oz. glasses of water each day to avoid dehydration and constipation He also recommended daily intake of nutrients through a good multi-vitamin supplement. Finally, Dr. Atkins mentioned getting plenty of exercise to speed weight loss.

Expected Results

You'll lose five pounds in your first week and then lose one to two pounds each week after that. Atkins and other low-carb diets have been studied longer and harder than most other approaches, and Atkins does appear to be moderately successful, especially in the first couple of weeks.

That's only part of the story, however. Much of the initial loss is water, say experts, because of the diet's diuretic effect. That's true of many other diets, too, and is one of the reasons researchers don't judge diets based on a few weeks of results. In diet studies, long-term generally starts at two years.

Health risks/ Dangers

No indications of serious short-term risks have surfaced. Reported side effects are generally minor. They include weakness, nausea, dizziness, constipation, irritability, and bad breath. However, long-term risks are uncertain.

Most experts feel that diets high in saturated fat significantly raise the risk of heart disease and cardiovascular events such as heart attack and stroke. The latest Atkins book calls this a "myth," however, asserting that carb restriction changes the way the body processes fat in the diet.

Keep in mind Atkins isn't safe for everyone. Pregnant women should go directly to the phase 4 maintenance stage. Adolescents and diabetics on medications to control blood sugar should consult with their doctors.

How Easy It Is to Follow

The diet is quite strict and bans the entire groups of foods for months or even years. For instance, if you are a big fan of bread, pizzas, pastas, etc., it will be pretty hard for you to follow it.

If you are eating at home, it may be not that easy to cook by yourself the foods suggested by the Atkins diet, as well as going out makes it also quite difficult to follow the diet. Also, the consumption of alcohol is limited. Several years ago, in 2013, Atkins presented the line of frozen food, which is the first low-carb frozen food line on the market, so it may be helpful for you as well.

Atkins provides meal plans and recipes with the lists of ingredient, food carb counts. The choice of recipes is pretty large and offers a variety of choices – from American to Asian cuisines, so everyone can actually find a right match for himself.

During the Phase 1, you have to exclude the alcohol from your menu completely. So if you've got used to having a beer or a glass of wine while having your meal, it may be a bit more complicated to follow the diet. On the Phase 2 it is allowed to have maximum one drink per day. However, the specialists claim that consumption of alcohol may influence the flow of the diet and make your weight loss process slower.

If you are in a hurry and don't have enough time to cook, there several meal options that you can purchase, such as shakes ($7 for a four-pack), snack bars ($6 for a five-pack), penne pasta ($4 for 12 ounces), and all-purpose baking mix ($10 for 2 pounds).

On its website, free meal planners and carb counter are available, as well as interactive goal-setting tools and discussion forums.

What also makes the diet easy to follow is that it includes a lot of protein and fat that generally take long time to digest. That's why at least two hours after having a meal; you will not feel hungry for sure, which is an advantage of the diet. Moreover, despite the diet has some restrictions, it also allows you to include into the menu quite a big variety of foods which taste really good, so another positive thing about the Atkins Diet is that it can be absolutely delicious!

Price/ Cost

Meat and fresh veggies are pricier than most processed and fast foods. How much more you'll spend will depend largely on your choices of protein sources. Are you buying mostly ground beef or springing for veal? Chicken or turkey? Chuck vs. New York strip? Buying in season should keep the veggie tab reasonable. *The New Atkins for a New You*, an essential guide, is $16.

3. *South Beach*

Ranking: 3.0 out of 5.0

How Long It's Been Around

Arthur Agatston, the originator of the South Beach diet, is a medical doctor. He is has a cardiology practice that emphasizes disease prevention and is an associate professor at the University of Miami Miller School of Medicine in Miami, Florida.

In 2003, he published The South Beach Diet: The Delicious, Doctor-designed, Foolproof Plan for Fast and Healthy Weight Loss. Television coverage boosted the popularity of the South Beach diet, and in 2004, Kraft Foods entered into an agreement that allowed it to use the South Beach diet name on line of foods that were nutritionally compatible with the diet.

How It Works

The South Beach diet is part a fast-weight-loss diet and part a calorie-restricted, portion-controlled long-term diet. The diet unfolds in three "phases," but if you have less than 10 pounds to lose, you can start with phase 2. Each phase becomes progressively less restrictive.

The focus is on replacing bad carbs with good carbs and bad fats with good fats. There's no counting calories, fat grams, carbohydrates, or anything else. You'll eat three meals a day, plus two snacks, and one high-protein dessert (like maple-almond flan or creamy chocolate mousse). The diet lasts as long as you want—it depends on your weight-loss goal.

Phase 1, the shortest and most restrictive, lasts two weeks and is intended to stabilize blood sugar and eliminate cravings. You'll eat generous portions of lean protein (fish, shellfish, chicken, turkey, and soy); lots of vegetables, salads, beans, eggs, and low-fat dairy; and up to 2 tablespoons a day of healthy fats, such as nuts and extra-virgin olive oil.

You won't touch fruit, fruit juice, starches (including pasta, rice, and bread), whole grains, sugary foods, or alcohol. "The South Beach Diet Supercharged," by South Beach creator and cardiologist Arthur Agatston, provides a detailed list of what you can and cannot eat. Among the guidelines: Eat 4½ cups of vegetables and 2 cups of milk or dairy each day. Daily protein is unlimited. Even though phase 1 may melt off pounds, dieters are advised not to stay on it more than two weeks because it's so restrictive.

In phase 2, you'll reintroduce "good carbs," like whole-grain bread, brown rice, whole-wheat pasta, and fruit. You'll have three servings of fruit and three servings of starches a day. The two daily snacks required in phase 1 are now optional, but encouraged; a glass of red or white wine with dinner is OK. You'll stick with this phase until you reach your weight goal.

Phase 3, the maintenance phase, is your lifelong healthy way to eat. No food is off-limits. Guidelines advise eating 3 pieces of fruit a day, 3 to 4 servings of starches, and no more than 2 tablespoons of good fats, such as mayonnaise or margarine.

Expected Results

Most people lose 8 to 13 pounds within the first two weeks, the company says, though that number could be smaller depending on your start weight. From there on out, you'll drop 1 to 2 pounds a week.

What little research there is on South Beach does suggest it's an effective way to lose weight, at least in the short term. But whether it keeps the weight off long-term is unproven.

Because South Beach incorporates the glycemic index, encouraging only "good" carbs when they're allowed back in—it's worth considering research that suggests low-GI plans yield short-term weight loss (though not much more effectively than other approaches).

In 2009, the independent, nonprofit Cochrane Collaboration reviewed six small, randomized controlled trials of low-GI diets. Overall low-GI dieters fared slightly better than comparison dieters, losing an average of about 2 pounds more. That was a statistically significant difference, however.

Health risks/ Dangers

No indications of serious short-term risks or side-effects have surfaced. However, South Beach isn't safe for everyone.

Children should steer clear; weight-loss diets often aren't appropriate for kids, who need adequate calories and nutrients to grow.

Phase 1 is inappropriate for pregnant women, who need ample calories and nutrients. Losing too much weight too quickly also can harm a baby's health and development. But since South Beach is a lifestyle eating plan, pregnant women can go directly to phase 2, which encourages healthy eating choices. They should take in an additional three to four cups of fat-free or low-fat milk a day to provide the fetus with calcium and other nutrients.

Nursing mothers should start with phase 2, making sure to eat two to three servings of fruits and starches every day. But they should aim to lose no more than one pound per week. Any more is unsafe, since ample nutrients and calories are required to successfully breastfeed, the company says. Besides, a nursing mother is already burning an extra 200 to 500 calories daily.

How Easy It Is to Follow

The strictest phase of the South Beach diet lasts only for two weeks. However, even after that you have to exclude from your menu such products as bread, honey, sweets, etc. You will also have to limit in your daily ration such fruits as pineapple, raisins, watermelon, since they contain a lot of sugar. Alcohol is prohibited during phase 1 and limited during phase 2. Eating out and restaurants are allowed, as long as you follow the diet's rules and restrictions.

The detailed recipes with description and lists of ingredients, calorie counts, and nutritional facts are available online, as well as in a printed version, in "The South Beach Diet Super Quick Cookbook" ($28.99), one of six cookbooks that were published in 2010. "The South Beach Diet Gluten Solution Cookbook" ($27.99) was published in 2013.

Alcohol is forbidden during the first two weeks of the diet. After that, it is allowed to have one glass per day for women, and maximum two glasses – for men. The best choice would be a red wine, since it contains an antioxidant that can reduce heart risk.

In order to save time, South Beach offers a line of snack and meal bars, treats and ready-to-go smoothies. It includes cereal bars, 100-calorie snack bars, snack-sized smoothies, high-protein and meal bars, and gluten-free bars, which are free of artificial sweeteners, sugar and other flavors.

If you become an online member, you will get an opportunity to track meals, weight, and diet goals. Moreover, you can connect with other dieters through the company's forums and discussions. You can also subscribe to the regular newsletters that include tips on the diet, nutrition and healthy living generally.

Another good thing that makes the diet quite easy to follow is that you will not feel the hunger. The diet requires at least two snacks per day. Also, it includes foods that are fiber-packed, which promote fullness. And the best part of it is the fact that the diet is really tasty, so you will not only feel full, but also satisfied with the taste of your food.

During the phase 1 you will have to limit yourself more, and exclude form your menu some foods, but after that you will be more flexible and may allow yourself even sweets, pizzas and other culinary delicacies.

Price/ Cost

"The South Beach Diet Supercharged: Faster Weight Loss and Better Health for Life," an essential manual, costs $24.95. Optional online membership is $4 to $5 a week (the first seven days are free).

You'll get customized tools like a weight-loss tracker, a printable shopping list generator, daily newsletter, and access to community message boards and hundreds of recipes. Following the program's recommended meal plans to a T, however, could break the bank, with skillet pork chops on the menu one day and spicy shrimp stir-fry the next. You can make the diet more affordable with an online tool that helps customize meal plans to conform to your budget.

4. Paleo

Ranking: 2.0 out of 5.0

How Long It's Been Around

The idea of a paleolithic diet can be traced to the work in the 1970s by gastroenterologist Walter Voegtlin. The idea was later developed by Stanley Boyd Eaton and Melvin Konner, and popularized by Loren Cordain in his 2002 book *The Paleo Diet*. The terms caveman diet and stone-age diet are also used, as is Paleo Diet, trademarked by Loren Cordain.

In 2012 the paleolithic diet was described as being one of the "latest trends" in diets, based on the popularity of diet books about it; in 2013 the diet was Google's most searched-for weight-loss method.

How It Works

The paleolithic diet is a diet based on the food humans' ancient ancestors might likely have eaten, such as meat, nuts and berries,[1] and excludes food to which they had not yet become familiar, like dairy. The Paleolithic era was a period lasting around 2.5 million years that ended about 10,000 years ago with the advent of farming. It was characterized by the use of flint, stone, and bone tools, hunting, fishing, and the gathering of plant foods.

The diet is based on the premise that Paleolithic humans evolved nutritional needs specific to the foods available at that time, and that the nutritional needs of modern humans remain best adapted to the diet of their Paleolithic ancestors.

Proponents argue that this is because modern human metabolism has been unable to adapt fast enough to handle many of the foods that have become available since the advent of agriculture. Thus, modern humans are said to be maladapted to eating foods such as grain, legumes, and dairy, and in particular the high-calorie processed foods that are a staple of most modern diets.

Proponents claim that modern humans' inability to properly metabolize these comparatively new types of food has led to modern-day problems such as obesity, heart disease, and diabetes. They claim that followers of the

Paleolithic diet may enjoy a longer, healthier, more active life.

Critics of the Paleolithic diet have raised a number of objections, including that paleolithic humans did eat grains and legumes, that humans are much more nutritionally flexible than Paleolithic advocates claim, that Paleolithic humans were not genetically adapted to specific local diets, that the Paleolithic period was extremely long and saw a variety of forms of human sustenance, or that little is known for certain about what Paleolithic humans ate.

Expected Results

Paleo is not a weight-loss "diet." It's a way of eating for health and longevity – which, for some people, involves weight loss as one piece of the big picture.

Weight loss does not look like a straight line down from your starting weight to your goal weight. Wouldn't we all love that! Instead, here's what to expect for the first few weeks. Initially, most people see a very rapid loss of 5-10 pounds in the first week. This is encouraging, but don't expect it to last forever: it's mostly water weight. Why so much water weight? Every gram of glucose (carbohydrate) in your body holds on to 3-4 grams of water. So when you lower carbohydrate intake, you're losing a whole lot of water weight along with the carbs. This isn't good or bad; it's just a physiological effect of lowering carbs. After the initial dramatic dip, weight loss continues at a slow and steady pace.

Health risks/ Dangers

There are no significant risks identified with the Paleo diet. However, the Paleo diet has some flaws. The evolutionary arguments don't hold up, and the evidence for excluding dairy, legumes, and grains isn't strong yet.

How Easy It Is to Follow

Paleo diet restricts entire food groups, which makes it quite difficult to follow. You will have to get used to the idea of breadless sandwiches and having your milk and cookies without either milk or cookies. But nobody said you can not allow yourself to have a cheat meal! Sometimes.

You can find plenty of recipes at several thematic web-pages, such as like Paleo Diet Lifestyle. There's even "The

Paleo Diet Cookbook," "Everyday Paleo" and "The Primal Blueprint Cookbook." Eating out may be quite problematic for Paleo dieters, since not all of cafes or restaurants serve the food acceptable for the diet. However, the solution can be to order lean meat or sea food with vegetables, and some fruits for the dessert.

Alcohol is forbidden in the true Paleo diet. But occasionally you can allow yourself to have a drink or two, for example, as a part of your cheat meal.

"The Paleo Diet" offers sample meal plans and recipes, lists of approved foods and also some practical tips and advices how to follow the diet in the most effective way when you, for example, travelling or eating out. The diet consists of a lot of food with protein and fiber that are quite filling, so you will not feel hungry, and this is a big advantage of the Paleo diet.

Price/ Cost

It may be pricey – the produce section and meat counter are among the priciest corners of the grocery store.

5. *Mediterranean Diet*

Ranking: 3.9 out of 5.0

How Long It's Been Around

The origins of the pattern of food consumption found in Mediterranean countries go back several millennia into history; descriptions of meals in ancient Greek and Roman literature would not be out of place in contemporary Mediterranean diet cookbooks.

The first description of the traditional Mediterranean diet as it was followed in the mid-twentieth century, however, was not in a cookbook; it was in a research study funded by the Rockefeller Foundation and published in 1953. The author was Leland Allbaugh, who carried out a study of the island of Crete as an underdeveloped area.

Allbaugh noted the heavy use of olive oil, whole-grain foods, fruits, fish, and vegetables in cooking as well as the geography and other features of the island.

How It Works

The Mediterranean diet is better described as a nutritional model or pattern of food consumption rather than a diet in the usual sense of the word.

In general, Mediterranean diets have five major characteristics:

— High levels of fruits and vegetables, breads and other cereals, potatoes, beans, nuts, and seeds.

— Olive oil as the principal or only source of fat in the diet.

— Moderate amounts of dairy products, fish, and poultry; little use of red meat.

— Eggs used no more than 4 times weekly.

— Wine consumed in moderate amounts—two glasses per day for men, one glass for women.

Since wine and olive oil are obtained from their respective plant sources by physical (crushing or pressing) rather than chemical processes, their nutrients retain all the properties of their sources. Wine contains polyphenols, which are powerful antioxidants and also have a relaxing effect on blood vessels, thus lowering blood pressure.

Expected Results

This diet scores big for heart health. Studies suggest it can make you less likely to get heart disease, lower your blood pressure and cholesterol, and may also help you avoid certain cancers and chronic diseases.

For weight loss, you'll have better results if you stick with it more than six months, get regular exercise, and cut back on how much you eat. Studies show it may be better for weight loss than a low-fat diet.

Health risks/ Dangers

There are no major risks associated with following a traditional Mediterranean diet for people who have consulted a physician beforehand if they intend to use the diet as a weight-loss regimen. Health crises caused by food interactions with MAOIs are uncommon but can be fatal (about 90 deaths over a 40-year period).

The risk of cancer or any other disease from aflatoxin-contaminated olive oil is minimal in the United States and Canada.

How Easy It Is to Follow

It's a tasty and good for you, though you may have a learning curve at first. The Mediterranean diet has very few limitations, so it allows plenty of variety and experimentation. A lot of inspiration and healthy recipes can be found in "The New Mediterranean Diet Cookbook: A Delicious Alternative for Lifelong Health."

Eating out shouldn't be a problem, since you can always go for salads, vegetables, fish and other foods that are allowed according to the diet. As an option, you can always share the meal with a friend, but most of the restaurants will definitely have in their menus something for you.

If you ask about alcohol, the answer would be simple. Can you imagine the Mediterranean diet without wine? Of course, no, since this is an important part of the culture and, we can even say, the essential part of the daily menu. So it is allowed to have a glass of wine for women, and two glasses – for men. Red wine would be the best choice, since it is known for its good influence on health and general well-being.

Another positive thing about the diet is that you shouldn't have any problems with feeling full, since the fiber is filling, and you'll be eating lots of fiber-packed produce and whole grains. And it can taste really, really good, if you make an effort and dedicate some time for searching for recipes and cooking. Since there is no any time-savers, you are responsible for your food and how it tastes, so make it good!

Price/ Cost

It's moderately pricey. While some ingredients (olive oil, nuts, fish and fresh produce in particular) can be expensive, you can find ways to keep the tab reasonable. Good wine you can find for nearly $15. And snag whatever veggies are on sale that day, rather than the $3-a-piece artichokes.

6. *Mayo Clinic Diet*

Ranking: 3.9 out of 5.0

How Long It's Been Around

The Mayo Clinic Diet is a diet created by Mayo Clinic. Prior to this, use of that term was generally connected to fad diets which had no association with Mayo Clinic. The diet developed and endorsed by Mayo Clinic is presented in the form of a book, The Mayo Clinic Diet and a logbook, The Mayo Clinic Diet Journal.

The Mayo Clinic fad diet is believed to date back to the 1930s, when it was known as the Hollywood diet. It may be that the public thought that following the diet would quickly lead a dieter to have a slender figure like those of the movie stars.

How It Works

This diet begins with a two-week period where five specific bad habits are replaced by five specific good habits. As we've already mentioned before, the diet consists of two phases:

Phase 1: Lose It! It is designed to jump-start your weight loss and help you lose up to 6 to 10 pounds in two weeks in a safe and healthy way. You'll learn how to add good habits to help you succeed; plus, you'll discover which bad habits are sabotaging your diet.

Phase 2: Live It! will help you continue to lose 1 to 2 pounds a week until you reach your goal weight. After that, you'll get expert guidance and techniques to help you maintain your weight loss for life. This is designed to be the last diet you'll ever need.

The program uses a food pyramid that has vegetables and fruits as its base. It puts carbohydrates, meat and dairy, fats, and sweets into progressively more limited daily allowances. The diet emphasizes setting realistic goals, replacing poor health habits with good ones, and conscious portion control.

Expected Results

The primary benefit of the Mayo Clinic fad diet is that a person quickly loses weight. For some people, a diet of several weeks is easier to follow than one that could last months or one described as a lifetime of healthy eating. On the fad plan, dieters do not have to count calories or track the fat and fiber of content of foods. People follow a plan consisting of several basic foods. The diet is more affordable than some weight-loss plans that require the purchase of meals.

Furthermore, dieters could feel that they aren't depriving themselves because they're allowed to eat as much as they want of meat and other high-fat proteins. People fond of fried foods will be happy that they don't have to give up those items.

The plan consists of a limited selection of food so it will be easy for dieters to shop and to know what to eat. While the repetitive nature of the diet may become monotonous, that sameness may help curb dieters' appetites. The monotony for some dieters is endured by the knowledge that the diet is short-term.

Health risks/ Dangers

Risks associated with the fad diet range from the medication-grapefruit interaction to the potential for complications related to a high-fat diet. The Mayo Clinic in 2006 cautioned that chemicals in grapefruit and grapefruit juice interfere with the body's process of breaking down drugs in the digestive system.

The interference could produce excessively high levels of the drug in the blood. The interaction could occur with some medications to treat high blood pressure, HIV, high cholesterol, arrhythmia (abnormal heart rhythm), and erectile dysfunction. There is also a potential for interaction with some anti-depressants, anti-seizure medications, tranquilizers, immunosuppressant drugs and the pain relief drug Methadone.

People with concerns about grapefruit should ask their physician or pharmacist about possible drug interactions or alternative medications.

When the person ends the diet and again eats carbohydrates, the body responds by converting food into fat. This protection against starvation results in a weight gain.

How Easy It Is to Follow

The first phase "Lose it!" may be quite difficult to follow. The good news is that lasts for two weeks only, so if you are having a strong will, it is more than possible to go through it. Once you develop your plan in "Live it!" and find no foods completely off limits, you'll be more likely to stay on the track.

Eating out may be problematic on the first phase of the diet, since it is quite strict. But on the second phase, if you follow the pyramid and stay on your eating plan, eating out actually becomes possible.

Alcohol is also not allowed during "Lose it!" and should be considered a treat in "Live it!" with no more than 500 calories from alcohol per week.

Also, you shouldn't feel hungry on the Mayo Clinic Diet. During the first part of the diet, you can snack on unlimited veggies and fruits, and later, the emphasis on low-energy-dense fruits, veggies and high-fiber whole grains should keep you feeling fuller longer.

How delicious your food is going to be, depends on you, since you cannot buy already prepared food or use any other time-savers, and have to plan and cook by yourself (or hire someone who will do it instead of you).

Price/ Cost

Whether it's pricier than your current grocery tab depends, of course, on what you put in your cart. Fruits, veggies and whole-grain products are generally more expensive than sugary cereal, white bread and frozen pizzas.

But there's no membership fee, and the diet's individualized nature gives you financial wiggle room – by making dinner from whatever produce is on sale, for example. The *"Mayo Clinic Diet"* book, an essential guide, is $26.

7. DASH Diet

Ranking: 4.1 out of 5.0

How Long It's Been Around

DASH stands for the Dietary Approaches to Stop Hypertension. The DASH diet is based on DASH Study results published in 1997.

How It Works

The diet is based on 2,000 calories with the following nutritional profile:

— Total fat: 27% of calories

— Saturated fat: 6% of calories

— Protein: 18% of calories

— Carbohydrate: 55% of calories

— Cholesterol: 150mg

— Sodium: 2,300 mg

— Potassium: 4,700 mg

— Calcium: 1,250 mg

— Magnesium: 500 mg

— Fiber: 30 g

These percentages translate into more practical guidelines using food group servings which are available in the National Institutes of Health (NIH) updated booklet *"Your Guide to Lowering Your Blood Pressure with DASH"*, which also provides background information, weekly menus, and recipes.

The Dash diet was not designed for weight loss but it can be adapted for lower calorie intakes. The NIH booklet provides guidelines for a 1,600-calorie diet. Vegetarians can also use the diet, as it is high in fruits, vegetables, beans, seeds, and low-fat dairy, which are the main sources of protein in a vegetarian diet. The DASH meal plan is a healthy diet recommended for those with and without high blood pressure.

Expected Results

The DASH diet may lower blood pressure as much as taking medication, but without the risk of unwanted side effects. The dietary changes can also have immediate effects comparable with drug therapy. A blood pressure reduction of the degree seen in the DASH study is estimated to reduce the incidence of coronary artery disease by 15% and stroke by 27%.

Health risks/ Dangers

Currently, there are no known risks associated with the DASH diet. However, the long-term effects of the diet on morbidity and mortality are still unknown.

How Easy It Is to Follow

The DASH diet doesn't restrict entire groups of foods, so it relatively easy to follow, even though you may miss your favorite sweets, or other fatty, sugary and salty products.

Eating out may be difficult, since very often meals that are served in restaurants are oversized, with a lot of salt and fat. Pay attention to the menu, choose fruits and vegetables, or as an option, ask a chef to change the way of seasoning the meal. Too much of alcohol can elevate blood pressure and damage the liver, brain and heart. Following the DASH diet, moderation is the key. One drink a day for women, and two a day for men are still fine.

DASH foods lean protein and fiber-filled fruits and veggies, so you will not feel hungry, which is a good thing about this diet. You may miss the taste of salty food, but after some time, your body and taste sensors will adjust.

Price/ Cost

Fresh fruits, veggies and whole-grain products are generally pricier than the processed, fatty, sugary foods most Americans consume.

8. *TLC Diet*

Ranking: 4.0 out of 5.0

How Long It's Been Around

TLC diet, Therapeutic Lifestyle Changes diet is designed by National Cholesterol Education Program (NECP) to lower your cholesterol by regulating your diet to elevate your physical activity, reduce weight and threats of heart attacks. Although, the diet is not designed to cut down weight, it is well-liked, as it not only helps in weight loss but is also good for overall health.

The National Institutes of Health created the National Cholesterol Education Program in 1985 to reduce cardiovascular disease rates in the United States by addressing high cholesterol.

They created the TLC diet to be used alone or in conjunction with medication management to control elevated cholesterol. The diet was incorporated into the Adult Treatment Panel III (ATP III) for high cholesterol in adults which was released in 2002. Updated guidelines for cholesterol management were established in 2013 by the

American Heart Association (AHA) and American College of Cardiology (ACC).

How It Works

The three cornerstones of the TLC lifestyle modification diet are:

Dietary Changes. Reduction of saturated fat, trans-fat, and cholesterol within the diet. Addition of plant stanols and sterols. Increased consumption of soluble fiber.

Weight Management. Weight loss can help lower LDL and is especially important for those with a cluster of risk factors that includes high triglyceride and/or low HDL levels. For those with a large waist measurement (more than 40 inches for men and more than 35 inches for women) it is important to lose weight to decrease the risk for developing heart disease.

Physical Activity. Regular physical activity, at least 30 minutes on most, if not all, days is recommended every day of the week. Physical activity can help raise HDL and lower LDL and is important for those with high triglyceride and/or low HDL levels who are overweight with a large waist measurement

The TLC eating plan is one that advises less than 7% of calories from saturated fat and less than 200 mg of dietary cholesterol per day. There should be no more than 25-35% or less of total daily calories coming from total fat intake. A limit of 2400 mg of day of sodium is recommended.

The TLC diet recommends weight maintenance and avoidance of weight gain through caloric homeostasis. If LDL cholesterol is not lowered through reduction of saturated fat and cholesterol intakes, then it is suggested that the amount of soluble fiber in the diet be increased.

The TLC Program is adjusted using a set of four categories that are based on ones heart disease risk profile to set LDL goals and treatment steps. For a person who has heart disease or diabetes, they are considered a category I, carrying the highest risk. For persons free of those conditions, their needs are based upon their personal risk of having a heart attack in the next 10-years based upon the Framingham Heart Study.

The higher a person's risk category, the more important it is for them to lower their LDL and control any other heart disease risk factors (including smoking and high blood pressure) they have.

Expected Results

TLC diet is not designed for losing weight, but for lowering cholesterol levels. Thus, it is not entirely suitable for people seeking to shed weight, even though it does result in weight-loss to some extent. However, it should not be taken primarily for this purpose. However, it is healthy and brings about positive changes in lifestyle, as it helps in lowering cholesterol levels and high blood pressure.

Health risks/ Dangers

According to the NCEP Guidelines, all adults 20 years of age and older should have their total cholesterol as well as HDL-cholesterol measured every five years.

How Easy It Is to Follow

The TLC diet is simple, straightforward and quite easy to follow. Eating out is allowed, but you have to be careful with the menu and choose foods with the low level of saturated fat and cholesterol. Smartest are steamed, broiled, baked, roasted or poached entrees.

The consumption of alcohol should be limited as well, but one drink per day for women or two drinks for men are acceptable. Since the diet includes a lot of fiber-packed fruits and veggies, you shouldn't feel hungry. But if you are a big fan of fast food, sweets, butter, etc., you do may miss these products, but only in the beginning. After some time, you will definitely get used to the new ration.

Price/ Cost

Other than your grocery bill, which should be no higher than usual, there are no expenses.

9. Weight Watchers

Ranking: 3.9 out of 5.0

How Long It's Been Around

By the mid-2000s, more than 25 million people worldwide had participated in the Weight Watchers program that was started in the living room of an overweight housewife in Queens, New York. When Jean Nidetch needed to lose weight, she attended a diet clinic sponsored by the New York City Board of Health.

However, after she had lost about 20 lb (10 kg), she found it hard to remain motivated to stay on the diet. Her solution was to ask a group of overweight friend to come to her house and talk about their eating and dieting challenges. This group evolved into a regular support group. While attending this group, Nidetch had the insight that dieting was not just about food, but about changing behaviors.

Two years later in 1963, Nidetch established Weight Watchers as a company and held her first public meeting. Demand for her program far exceeded expectations. Over the years the program evolved to incorporate new research in nutrition. Behavior management modules and an exercise program were added. In 1978 the company was bought by H. J. Heinz Company, which added a line Weight Watchers supermarket foods.

Today Weight-Watcher endorsed cookbooks, exercise tapes, and a magazine all are available to support dieters who are either Weight Watcher members or who want to try the diet plan on their own.

How It Works

Weight Watchers is the largest commercial weight-loss program in the world. The diet is based on calorie and portion control while eating regular food, exercise, and behavior modification.

The fundamental message of the Weight Watcher program is "move more, eat less." There is nothing unique about this approach to dieting. What distinguishes the Weight Watchers program are the tools it provides members to stay motivated to meet these goals.

Weight Watchers diet plans have evolved over the years. The current system gives a choice of two plans, he Flex

Plan or the Core Plan. The Flex Plan assigns a point value per serving to every food. Points are based on the amount of calories, dietary fiber, and fat in the food. The Core Plan gives dieters a list of "core foods."

They may eat unlimited quantities (within reason) of any of the core foods without weighing or measuring. Motivation is a big part of the Weight Watchers program. At every in-person meeting, the member is privately weighed and their weight recorded. Even small successes are celebrated. Daily exercise is strongly encouraged at Weight Watchers, but it is not a required part of the program.

Expected Results

The diet plan is designed for slow, steady weight loss of between 1.5 and 2 pounds per week.

Health risks/ Dangers

Individuals who are under treatment for an illness, taking prescription drugs, or on a therapeutic diet (e.g. low sodium, gluten-free) should consult their doctor about the Weight Watchers plan and follow any changes or modifications the physician makes to the Weight Watchers plan. Failure to do this can increase the risk of developing health complications.

How Easy It Is to Follow

You menu is based on points that you are collecting. For sure, it will be enough to have three meals and at least two snacks, so you will not be hungry following the Weight Watchers programme.

Moreover, the members are also given an extra 49 points a week to spend on "indulgences". reating You will be encouraged to treat yourself, and popular food choices include pasta, black bean soup and filet mignon. You don't have to worry about calculating points; it is pretty simple, wherever you are, at home, on the street or in the restaurant.

For this, you can use a pocket guide, pocket calculator and a PointsPlus application, which is available for iPhone and Android. The members of Weight Watchers programme can access thousands of free recipes on the website of the company (including lists of ingredients, description of preparation process, points, etc.).

For eating out, it is recommended to take with you the Weight Watchers "Dining Out Companion," which serves up the nutritional low-down on meals at hundreds of restaurants, and includes tips on how to make your visits to the restaurants healthier.

You also don't have to exclude alcohol, but you do have to consume it moderately. For alcoholic drinks, you can spend some points, but then you will have less of them for food, so basically, it's your choice.

The members of Weight Watchers programme can also access weight-tracking tools, fitness tips, workout video demonstrations and restaurant guides on the website of the company.

The program emphasizes fiber-packed Power Foods, which will keep you feeling fuller, so you will not feel hungry.

Besides that, you will have 49 extra points weekly, which you will be able to spend for some additional snacks, if for one or another reason you are not feeling full. And what is really good about the Weight Watchers is that you don't have to exclude your favorite foods from your menu, even if it is a double-cheese pizza. The diet simply helps you to control portions and tweak your favorite recipes making them healthier.

Price/ Cost

Cost varies with promotions throughout the year and depending on whether you choose to attend weekly in-person meetings, work with a coach, use the online tools only or all three.

All new members pay a $20 starter fee plus a standard monthly fee of at least $19.95 for essentials including the online tools and 24/7 chat. You can add to that a monthly pass to unlimited in-person meetings for $44.95, which also includes the essentials. Or you can pay as you go; meetings are $12 to $15 per week, with a one-time $20 registration fee. For a personal coach (plus essentials), members pay $54.95 a month. If you want "total access" – meetings and a virtual coach, plus essentials – you pay $69.95 each month. None of the costs include food.

10. Jenny Craig

Ranking: 3.7 out of 5.0

How Long It's Been Around

Jenny Craig and her husband Sig Craig founded Jenny Craig Weight Management Program in Australia in 1983. The program has since expanded to the United States, Canada, New Zealand, and Puerto Rico and offers both a center-based program and an at-home program.

Craig, who has no training as a nutritionist, based her program on her own successful experience with personalized weight loss. The program has a medical advisory board consisting of at least one physician, nutritionist, and behaviorist.

How It Works

Jenny Craig has quite the diet package, and we're not just talking about the food. With this plan, you'll get prepackaged low-calorie food, a consultant to offer support in person or on the phone (if you want), online tools to help you plan and track meals, and an exercise plan.

There are no banned foods, "detox" potions, or menus loaded with exotic foods that claim to melt fat. You'll mostly eat Jenny Craig's weekly menus of 70 different prepackaged foods, at least at first. You'll get about 1,200 calories a day, depending on your height and weight.

Besides Jenny Craig prepackaged meals, you can also have fresh fruits and vegetables, and reduced-fat dairy products. Jenny Craig's approach focuses on choosing low-fat foods that are rich in water, fiber, and protein to fill you up. In general, you can eat as many non-starchy vegetables (like tomatoes, broccoli, and peppers) as you want. No food is ever completely off-limits.

Expected Results

Jenny Craig promises dieters that if they follow her program, they will lose 1-2 pounds or 1% of their body weight weekly.

Once the weight-loss goal is met, a maintenance program is designed to solidify lifestyle changes and keep the weight off. Jenny Craig does not make any claims about the percentage of people who successfully keep weight off for an extended period.

Health risks/ Dangers

Meals on the Jenny Craig plan fall within the federal Dietary Guidelines for Americans 2005, and dietary supplements provided with the pre-packaged meals assure that the dieter of getting an adequate supply of vitamins and minerals.

The greatest risk to this diet program is that people do not learn how to shop and prepare healthy meals on their own. They lose weight eating the pre-packaged meals, but when they transition to the next stage of the diet, they go back to their old eating habits and gain the weight back. This type of weight cycling or yo-yo dieting can cause potential health problems.

How Easy It Is to Follow

The diet is easy to follow, first of all, because you don't have to worry about the menu, products and foods. There is nothing more convenient than having your meal delivered to your doorstep or just picked at a center.

The diet also allows the occasional restaurant meal, because sometimes you just can't avoid it, for example, meeting friends, having birthday parties, etc. If your dining out choice exceeds the calories for the menu you've preplanned with your consultant, you can compensate it with some extra exercising.

The book "Weight Loss Manual" is available, and it also offers tips for dining out, and other healthy advices that will make the flow of your diet much easier. Morcover, if needed, your consultant will help you to balance your ration.

Alcohol is not forbidden in this diet, but you have to limit yourself, especially in the beginning of your program. If you would like to have, for example, an extra glass of wine, you can skip two servings of fat that day, or make sure you cut out or burn off an additional 100 calories. The diet's approach involves choosing the least "energy-dense foods", so it guarantees feeling full for a longer time. Moreover, the Jenny's menu is low in fat and rich in water, fiber and protein which are the least energy-dense.

Price/ Cost

Jenny Craig is expensive enough to deter some dieters. To become a member, you pay a $99 enrollment fee and at least $19 a month for unlimited consultations. If you only want one consultation each week, you can pay $29 a month and skip the enrollment fee. But that doesn't include food, which costs an average of $15 to $23 each day. Tack on that shipping costs, if you plan to have your meals delivered.

11. Biggest Loser

Ranking: 3.6 out of 5.0

How Long It's Been Around

The programme is based on the approaches of the Biggest Loser, a reality television show which started in the U.S. in 2004. So in fact, you will train and eat like people on the NBC TV show The Biggest Loser, but without cameras following you around 24-7.

How It Works

Choosing healthy foods and getting lots of exercise is a winning combo. You can build strength, lose pounds, and be healthier. But be prepared to work hard and change your long-term eating and exercise habits.

You'll eat small, frequent meals. Most of your food is lean protein, low-fat dairy or soy, fruits, vegetables, whole grains, beans, and nuts. It's based on The Biggest Loser's 4-3-2-1 Pyramid: four servings of fruits and vegetables, three servings of lean protein, two servings of whole grains, and 200 calories of "extras."

Most foods are low in calories but high in fiber, to help you feel fuller longer.

By eating five to six small meals and snacks, you'll keep your blood sugar and hunger in check. The diet recommends drinking 6-8 glasses of water a day and avoiding caffeine.

Expected Results

By helping you lose weight, the diet may help lower your odds of getting type 2 diabetes, heart disease, high blood pressure, stroke, and certain cancers. The exercise is also good for you.

The program includes whole foods that are high in fiber and low in saturated fat and salt. The diet is in line with what most major health organizations recommend, including the American Heart Association.

Health risks/ Dangers

The Biggest Looser diet is generally considered to be safe, unless you are having individual reaction of the organism on a diet.

How Easy It Is to Follow

The Biggest Loser diet doesn't ban entire food groups, so it makes it quite easy to follow. You can find plenty of healthy recipes online, as well as in the Biggest Loser dietitian Cheryl Forberg's "Flavor First" cookbook

Eating out is allowed as long as you are making smart choices and break the diet's flow. You will have to avoid ordering pan-fried, grilled, steamed, baked, broiled or poached foods. Feel free to ask the chef to make some little changes in your meal, in order to make it healthy and acceptable for the diet.

Alcohol, as in any other diet, has to be limited, since it not only has a lot of calories, but also slows the fat-burning process and stimulating the appetite. However, one drink a day for women and two drinks a day for men is acceptable.

If you don't have time or wish to cook, you can purchase the Biggest Loser's "Simply Sensible" packaged entrees. There are also Biggest Loser-emblazoned bars, shakes, protein powder and cream of wheat, which you can order through eDiets.

However, it is recommended to cook by yourself and eat the prepared meals only in the exceptional situations, when it is really necessary. On this diet you shouldn't feel hungry, since a fiber- or protein-packed meal or snack comes every few hours, so it will make you full for some time, which makes the diet very convenient.

Price/ Cost

Fresh fruits, veggies, whole grains, and fish are generally more expensive than a cart full of sugary cereal, white bread and sweets. But you're not paying a membership fee, and you can tweak the suggested meal plans to bring the tab down – buy whatever produce is on sale that day at the grocery store, for example.

"The Biggest Loser: The Weight Loss Program to Transform Your Body, Health and Life" is $15.45 for paperback and $9.99 for the ebook edition.

12. Slim Fast

Ranking: 3.3 out of 5.0

How Long It's Been Around

Slim-Fast was started in 1977 as a product line of the Thompson Medical Company, founded in the 1940s by S. Daniel Abraham. Slim-Fast used the phrase "a shake for breakfast, a shake for lunch, then a sensible dinner" for many years to describe the use of the products within the Slim-Fast plan.

With the addition of snacks and an approach that allows for different calorie plans, the brand now advocates a more flexible system.

How It Works

The Slim-Fast of today is different than you may remember: Gone are the days of shakes alone. The plan promises you can drop pounds with tasty snacks, meal replacements (shakes or bars), and one sensible meal a day. Slim-Fast calls it the "3-2-1 Plan."

Every day, you eat two Slim-Fast meal replacements, three optional 100-calorie snacks (Slim-Fast snack bars, fruits, veggies, or even nuts), and one 500-calorie meal that you provide.

Meal replacements include six flavors of 200-calorie protein meal bars, 8 pre-made protein meal shakes, and six flavors of powdered protein shake mixes (to be mixed with skim milk). For 100-calorie snack options, choose among four different Slim-Fast snack bars, including peanut butter crunch and double-Dutch chocolate, or fruit (an orange, cherries, banana, grapes, or pear), carrot sticks, pistachios, pretzels, sorbet, or nonfat yogurt.

For the meal you provide, Slim-Fast recommends filling half of your plate with vegetables (such as green beans, carrots, eggplant, spinach, or broccoli); a quarter with lean protein (beef, poultry, pork, tofu, or fish); and the remaining quarter with starch (whole wheat pasta or bread, brown rice, potatoes, or corn). Nothing is totally off-limits with Slim-Fast, including alcohol. The Slim-Fast web site features recipes for alcoholic and nonalcoholic drinks made with its shakes.

Expected Results

The program says you can lose a safe 1 to 2 pounds per week on the plan that provides roughly 1200 calories a day.

Health risks/ Dangers

No indications of serious risks or side effects have surfaced. However, the diet is not always suitable for the people under the age of 18, pregnant or breast-feeding women. In such a case it is strongly recommended to consult with a doctor.

How Easy It Is to Follow

The diet is actually easy to follow, if you like the taste of the shakes, bars and meals that it offers. Even though it has a big variety of flavors, such as chocolate mint, peanut butter cappuccino delight, French vanilla and strawberries, not everyone is actually getting used to their taste.

That is why it may be quite hard to follow the diet, because only one homemade meal a day is allowed. It also provides a lot of recipes for those foods that you have to cook by yourself, with the rich variety of ingredients and different cuisines. Occasional eating out is allowed, but if instead of a Slim-Fast meal bar or shake you are taking a restaurant meal, try not to go over 300 calories for lunch, and 500 to 600 for dinner.

Alcohol is not recommended on the Slim-Fast diet, but from time to time you can allow yourself to have a drink, such as a glass of wine of hard liquors, which are low in calories. The Slim-Fast meal replacements contain protein and fiber content, so you will not feel hunger for up to four hours, which also an important argument when choosing a diet.

Price/ Cost

An eight-pack of shakes runs about $10, and five snack bars about $5. You can order online at sources like amazon.com and drugstore.com, or buy the products at most grocery and convenience stores. Free online registration allows access to hundreds of recipes, plus tools such as meal and activity trackers.

13. NutriSystem

Ranking: 3.2 out of 5.0

How Long It's Been Around

NutriSystem began in 1972 as a producer of a liquid protein diet, which it abandoned in 1978 as a result of competition from Slim-Fast, Carnation weight loss products, and other over-the-counter liquid diet drinks. NutriSystem then started a chain of 1,200 bricks-and-mortar weight loss centers roughly similar to Weight Watchers; dieters came to the centers in person to weigh in and then purchased prepackaged portion-controlled meals to take home.

The company went bankrupt in the early 1990s but reinvented itself in 1999 as an online meal delivery service.

As of the early 2000s, customers may order their monthly food assortments by telephone as well as online. Although a free weight loss counseling service is available by telephone or online chat, fewer than 20% of customers make use of it.

How It Works

To begin the program, the client either chooses one of the six programs online and continues to fill out the order form for their 28-day supply of prepackaged foods, or calls the company's toll-free number to order over the phone.

To complete the first order, the dieter selects one breakfast, one lunch, one dinner item, and one dessert (dessert choices include non-sweet snacks like pretzels or nacho chips) for each day of the 28-day package.

The total meal plan is designed around eating five times a day—three meals and two snacks. The NutriSystem foods do not require refrigeration; they are prepared by a ''soft canning'' process and can be stored at room temperature.

Some items, such as the snack bars and nacho chips, are ready to eat; the others are prepared on the stovetop or in a microwave oven. Some require the addition of hot water. There are at least 120 different items for the dieter to choose among in each program, with new items added from time to time.

In addition to such predictable standbys as cinnamon oatmeal, chocolate pudding, and tuna casserole, the food choices include thin crust pizza with cheese, pot roast, vegetarian chili, chicken cacciatore, fettucine Alfredo, and almond biscotti.

NutriSystem claims that its food selections are based on the glycemic index (GI), which measures foods by their effect on a person's blood sugar level within two hours after a meal. Foods ranked low on the GI index raise blood sugar levels slowly and gradually, thus allowing a dieter to feel satisfied for longer periods of time. The company advertises this aspect of the program as the ''Glycemic Advantage.''

The dieter's first order arrives with a ''Welcome Kit'' containing a meal planner, which outlines the meals and snacks and includes a daily food diary for keeping track of the dieter's consumption of fresh foods as well as the prepackaged items.

The Welcome Kit also explains the support services available, including online chat groups, classes, newsletters, and the ''Daily Dose Motivational Message'' as well as the option of one-on-one telephone contact with a counselor.

The daily cost of the three prepackaged meals and dessert is about $10, which means that the dieter must allow close to $300 per month for the NutriSystem program in addition to the cost of fresh dairy products and produce. As of early 2007, the company is offering 7 days' worth of meals with the first 28-day package. In addition, customers who choose the auto-delivery option for their second and subsequent deliveries get a 10-percent discount for each month they remain in the program.

Expected Results

You may lose up to five pounds in your first week of your diet, and after that lose one to two pounds each week.

Health risks/ Dangers

The NutriSystem program seems safe from a nutritional standpoint for most dieters who have had a medical checkup for previously undiagnosed conditions or food allergies. It does not depend on appetite suppressants, fasting, or other practices that may be dangerous to health.

How Easy It Is to Follow

The diet is simple and easy to follow, since the main entrées can be ordered online and you will get the pre-portioned meals delivered right to your doorstep, and you will know exactly what and when you have to eat. But at the same time, it makes it more difficult. It means that you will have to exclude as much as possible eating out, dining in the restaurants, etc.

So as long as you can control yourself, it actually works. Alcohol is discouraged as well, but occasionally, you may have a glass of beer or wine. However, if you decide to (or have to) eat out, the company provides a "dining out guide" with tips and recommendations on healthy eating categorized by cuisine such as Thai, Italian and French.

Hunger shouldn't be a problem. The entrées may look smaller than what you're used to, but they are full of protein and fiber-packed produce, so it will not make you feel hungry. When it comes to the taste, as the research shows, most of the clients are satisfied with it, so it also shouldn't make any difficulties in the general flow of the diet.

Price/ Cost

A 28-day "Select Plan," which includes 10 days of frozen meals and 18 days of pantry food, generally costs between $300 and $340. Pantry-only plans are slightly cheaper. Remember: You've still got a monthly grocery bill to add to that. Your tab will vary depending on what produce you buy (go for anything in-season) and your protein choices (chicken and turkey are generally pretty affordable).

Nutrisystem still may be a bargain compared to competitor Jenny Craig. Jenny Craig charges a registration fee on top of its meals, which generally run at least $100 a week.

14. Vegetarian Diet

Ranking: 4.1 out of 5.0

How Long It's Been Around

The vegetarian diet had been around since the vegetarianism itself started to exist. Nowadays, there are different variations of the diet, based on different approaches and scientific researches. However, the principle and the idea of the diet stay the same: to exclude from your menu animal products and generally eat healthy foods such as fruits and vegetables instead.

How It Works

First of all, you have to choose which kind of vegetarian you want to be. Most of people choose a lacto-ovo approach, which means they exclude from their menu meat, fish, and poultry, but they are still eating dairy products and eggs.

Meanwhile, lacto-vegetarians, also exclude from the ration eggs, and ovo-vegetarians exclude dairy products as well; vegans exclude all animal products.

During the vegetarian diet, you will naturally consume fewer calories daily. For example, your daily menu may include 2 cups of fruit; 2½ cups of vegetables; 3 cups of dairy, 6 "ounce-equivalents" of grains, and 5½ ounce-equivalents of protein.

On the internet there is a lot of literature about vegetarianism, measuring calories, cooking tips, etc. In any case, a vegetarian diet is a healthy way to meet your nutritional needs. You have to understand that it is not based only on raw vegetables.

If you start searching for recipes and ideas for meals, you will be surprised how big choices you have and how delicious it can be! So make researches, check the vegetarian menus in the restaurants, and be ready to make your own experiments!

Expected Results

Actually, all vegetarians eat less calories, weight less and have a lower body mass index. So during the vegetarian diet you will likely lose several pounds, and also fend off chronic diseases.

Health risks/ Dangers

There are no any particular health risks or dangers associated with the diet. However, each person's experience of vegetarianism is individual, so your body and organism can react in a different way. That's why before starting the diet, it is recommended to consult with a doctor.

How Easy It Is to Follow

If this diet is easy to follow or not, depends on how much you love meat. If you can normally live without it and not suffer seeing someone eating a juicy steak, vegetarian diet will not be a problem for you. But if you are a meat-lover, sometimes, especially in the beginning of the diet, you may face some difficulties, but rather psychological. So if you have a strong will and wish to follow the vegetarian diet, you will definitely succeed!

Another thing that makes the diet easy to follow is that you will always have a lot (we mean, really a lot) of options what to eat. First of all, there are thousands of recipes available online for free, so you can always get some ideas and inspiration, and it can be very delicious! Secondly, you can always go to any restaurant, since mostly everywhere the menu includes vegetarian meals.

However, be careful, since vegetarian doesn't always mean healthy and restaurants often have pretty huge portions. Alcohol is allowed as well, but you should remember that it has a lot of calories and is generally bad for your health. One drink a day for women and two drinks a day for men are acceptable.

Also, you shouldn't feel hungry between meals on the vegetarian diet, since it is built around fiber-packed vegetables, fruits, and whole grains, which will keep you full.

Price/ Cost

It's moderately pricey. Stocking up on produce and whole grains can get expensive, especially if you buy organic, but bypassing the butcher will help keep the tab reasonable. Plus, lacto-ovo vegetarian staples like eggs and beans are some of the most affordable choices at the supermarket.

15. Raw Food Diet

Ranking: 2.3 out of 5.0

How Long It's Been Around

Raw food has its origins in prehistory. As humans gradually developed tools and learned to control fire, a raw food diet gave way to a diet of cooked food. Modern interest in a raw food diet began in the 1930s. Ann Wigmore (1909–1994) was an early pioneer in using raw or "living" foods to detoxify the body. Herbert Shelton (1895–1985) was another early advocate of the health benefits of raw foods.

Raw food began to develop a more high-profile following in the 1990s, as celebrities such as Demi Moore and Woody Harrelson embraced a raw food diet, and in the 2000s raw food restaurants and cafes began showing up in some trendy urban areas, especially in Northern California.

How It Works

As you could guess from the name of the diet, you'll mostly be eating raw fruits, vegetables, and grains. The premise is that heating food destroys its nutrients and natural enzymes, which is bad because enzymes boost digestion and fight chronic disease.

In short: When you cook it, you kill it. Some raw foodists believe cooking makes food toxic. They claim that a raw food diet can clear up headaches and allergies, boost immunity and memory, and improve arthritis and diabetes.

Think uncooked, unprocessed, mostly organic foods. Your staples: raw fruits, vegetables, nuts, seeds, and sprouted grains. Some eat unpasteurized dairy foods, raw eggs, meat, and fish and there are some potential health risks associated with doing this. Your food can be cold or even a little bit warm, as long as it doesn't go above 118 degrees. You can use blenders, food processors, and dehydrators to prepare foods.

Expected Results

Raw foodists claim that the raw food diet offers the following benefits: weight control (it is difficult, if not impossible, to become obese on a raw food diet), increased energy, better digestion, a stronger immune system, more mental clarity and creativity, improved skin, a reduced risk of heart disease and other chronic diseases.

For the most part, these benefits are what followers of the raw food diet report rather than benefits proven by research that would be accepted by nutritionist and practitioners of conventional medicine.

Health risks/ Dangers

This interest in correct eating only becomes an eating disorder when the obsession interferes with relationships and daily activities.

For example, an orthorectic may be unwilling to eat at restaurants or friends' homes because the food is "impure" or improperly prepared. The limitations they put on what they will eat can cause serious vitamin and mineral imbalances.

Orthorectics are judgmental about what other people eat to the point where it interferes with personal relationships. They justify their fixation by claiming that their way of eating is healthy. Some experts believe orthorexia may be a variation of obsessive-compulsive disorder.

In addition potential psychological harm, without rigorous meal planning, raw foodists are at high risk of developing certain vitamin deficiencies, depending on whether they follow a vegan, vegetarian, or meat-eating raw food diet. Vegans are at highest risk. The most common deficiencies are of vitamin B12 and protein.

How Easy It Is to Follow

Raw Food diet may be one of the most difficult to follow. Firstly, because there is no a common belief or study that would prove that raw food is indeed more useful for a human. So wherever you go or whoever you ask (doctors, nutrition specialists, etc.) the opinions will be different, so this is only your decision if you are having this diet or not.

You may find a lot of raw food recipes on the internet, and very often they can be absolutely delicious and creative! Raw food diet doesn't necessary mean that you can only eat cold fresh vegetables (as many people imagine it), your menu may be pretty impressive!

However, eating out will become difficult, since not many restaurants serve raw food, and not all chefs understand the raw food dirt. As an option, you could order a salad, but the dressing might contain ingredients that aren't raw or natural, so bring your own. Speaking about alcohol, you may have a glass of wine, since it doesn't go through a heating process. But other drinks, for example beer, which is boiled, and liquor, which goes through a distillation process, you have to cut off from your ration.

Another advantage of a raw food diet is that hunger shouldn't be a problem. If you balance you menu smart, such foods as beans and other legumes, veggies and whole grains, are believed to take longer to digest, so they'll keep you feeling fuller longer.

Price/ Cost

A raw food diet can be pricey. Organic ingredients tend to cost more than other types, and not every grocery store carries a wide array of raw and organic products. Plus, you'll need appliances: High-end blenders range from $300 to $600, for example, and food processors capable of slicing, grating, and shredding can go for $700. Dehydrators cost about $100 to $200.

Conclusion

In this book you have learned the key facts on America's most popular fad diets. Having read and reviewed all this information, it's my hope that you are one step closer to choosing the perfect diet for you!

This author has had great success with *The Zone* diet in combination with a *Vegetarian* diet for several years now. The ratio of fat:protein:carbs that I have found most effective is 1g fat:2g protein:3g carbs. For what it's worth, you might start there if you are not sure what to try next.

Keep in mind that eating a diet rich in organic fruits and vegetables is always healthy. Despite the myriad of information out there on dieting, you can't go wrong with good old organic fruits and veggies. Add a little exercise and a proper amount of sleep, and you have the recipe for success.

If you liked this book, please consider posting an honest review on Amazon. This helps to support me and also provides invaluable feedback from you, the reader. Thanks for your time and best of luck in your dieting ventures!

www.ingramcontent.com/pod-product-compliance
Lightning Source LLC
Chambersburg PA
CBHW050423290526
45786CB00003B/1376